Matcha Green Te
How a Miraculous Green
Get In The Best Shaj
By. Shaahin Cheyene
http://www.matchapedia.com

DISCLAIMERS OF WARRANTY AND LIMITATION OF LIABILITY

This is provided by The Author and/or The Publisher on an "as is" and "as available" basis. The Author and/or The Publisher makes no representations or warranties of any kind, expressed or implied, as to the operation of this book or the information, content, materials, or products included on this book. You expressly agree that you use of this book is at your sole risk.

To the full extent permissible by applicable law, The Author and The Publisher disclaim all warranties, express of implied, including, but not limited to, implied warranties or merchantability and fitness for a particular purpose. The Author and/or The Publisher will not be liable for any damages of any kind arising from the use of this book, including, but not limited to direct, indirect, incidental, punitive, and consequential damages.

Certain state laws do not allow limitations on implied warranties or the exclusion or limitation of certain damages. If these laws apply to you, some or all of the above disclaimers, exclusions, or limitations may not apply to you, and you might have additional rights.

The ideas, concepts and opinions expressed herein are intended to be used for educational purposes only. The book and recipes are sold with the understanding that authors and publisher are not rendering medical advice of any kind, nor is the book intended to replace medical advice, nor to diagnose, prescribe or treat any disease, condition, illness or injury.

It is imperative that before beginning any diet or exercise program, including this program, you receive full medical clearance from a licensed physician.

Authors and publisher claim no responsibility to any person or entity for any liability, loss, or damage caused or alleged to be caused directly or indirectly as a result of the use, application or interpretation of the material in the books or information contained herein.

The Food and Drug Administration has not evaluated the statements contained in this book.

HEALTH SUPPLEMENTS DISCLAIMER

Matcha tea was designed for people who wish to supplement their normal diets with additional nutrients, some in amounts significantly higher than would be found in an ordinary diet. Matcha tea has been carefully chosen because scientific research studies have indicated that the nutrients might have a beneficial effect on one or more aspects of health by supporting the structure or function of certain cells within the body. Your decision to supplement your diet with Matcha tea or any nutritional supplements should be based on your own research and investigation or in consultation with your personal health care provider.

The National Library of Medicine provides access to a database of thousands of research studies, many of which were used to research this book. If you would like to obtain references to some of these studies in abstract form, you can do so by going to www.ncbi.nlm.nih.gov/entrez/query.fcgi and doing a simple search for the name of the nutrient. When doing so, bear in mind that when a particular study showed an improvement or change in a laboratory "value" suggesting that there might be a health benefit from that nutrient, it does not necessarily guarantee that supplementing your diet with that nutrient will actually improve your health. All scientists can do is measure, evaluate and predict based upon a narrowly defined experimental procedure. Ultimately, you must draw your own conclusion as to the efficacy of any nutrient. The Author and/or The Publisher's products are not intended to diagnose, treat, prevent, mitigate or cure any diseases. If you are pregnant, nursing or have a known medical condition, are under a physician's care or taking prescription medications, we suggest consulting with your health care provider before starting on any high-potency supplementation program.

WARNING: Matcha tea contains caffeine. If you are caffeine sensitive please ask your doctor before taking this or any caffeine containing product.

The Food and Drug Administration has not evaluated these statements.

The author and publisher believe to the best of their knowledge that the information contained herein are balanced, truthful and not misleading.

This information does not in any way promote a specific brand. Although quality of each product will vary, the information herein applies equally to all green tea around the world.

This book is not attached (by physical attachment or reference) to any dietary supplement's label or labeling but is a general reference guide for green tea.

*The only way to make sense out of change is to plunge
into it, move with it, and join the dance.*

–Alan Watts

Introduction

Somewhere in between the madness of launching a startup
business and building our first home together, my wife and I both
picked up the habit of drinking coffee. For me it was espresso, for
my wife it was the iced variety. All was good, until one day we both
started to notice the unfortunate effects on our adrenal glands and
digestion. As the acid from our morning coffees started to build up in
both of our stomachs, I raced to find an alternative to our beloved
morning ritual.

Yes, it's true that coffee certainly gave us that extra pick up we
needed. Yes, we loved the taste and aroma, not to mention how I
enjoyed drinking from those little espresso cups. But after some time
the side effects of coffee really started to get to us. I remember
thinking to myself, "There must be something better than this."

Searching intensively online and at the local health food store, I
found several varieties of tea that were available at the time. I tried
them all. I tried white teas, black teas, green teas, and all varieties of
tea products. But none seemed to quite do the trick. That is, until I
was introduced to Matcha tea. I ordered my first tin of Matcha tea
directly from Japan (pre-Fukashima nuclear meltdown) and was
delighted with the effects. Compared to other teas, Matcha is highest
in antioxidants. I then learned that one cup of Matcha can deliver as
many antioxidants as 10 cups of the other teas. What is more
amazing is that Matcha is rich in a neuroprotective amino acid
known as L-theanine, which for some reason seems to balance out
the effects of the caffeine. [1]

We have been drinking Matcha tea for several years now and
both genuinely believe that our lives have improved. Not only do we

---

[1] My Life with Tea, Andrew Weil http://www.drweil.com/drw/u/ART03093/My-Life-
With-Tea-Part-Two.html

believe this tea helps fight disease, curb sugar cravings, burn fat, relax the nerves, help us to think more clearly, and give a general sense of wellbeing, but it also allows us to take a moment to sit and slow the world around us. It is my hope that you will sit down with a cup of Matcha tea and read this book to discover the inner calm that can come when you sip tea and slow your world.

Video: Alan Watts on Tea

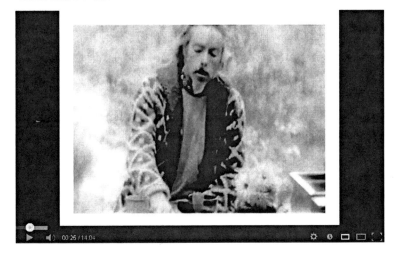

Contents

Chapter 1: History of Tea

Deep in China's Yellow River Valley, Emperor Cheng Tang sits nervously awaiting his medicine. The year is 1500 BC. The Shang Dynasty Emperor's personal physician has prepared a special medicinal drink. Rich in medicinal plants and herbs, the Yunnan region is known for its plant medicines.

The physician delivers the hot drink in a ceramic bowl. He gently whisks the powdered leaves in boiled water and nervously awaits the Emperor's verdict. Time stands still. The Emperor motions for another cup, and then another. After many hours and over 50 bowls of tea, the emperor finally looks up at the physician. He gently nods his head. It's a sign that he is in agreement. The drink is good. The Emperor is pleasantly surprised by its flavor and restorative properties. He declares the drink a magical royal elixir.

The drink is tea made from the leaves of the Camellia sinensis tree. Originating in Southeast Asia at the point of confluence of the lands of Northeast India, North Burma, Southwest China, and Tibet, the plant is quickly introduced to more than 52 countries. It quickly becomes known as a cultural staple, a sacred medicine, a commodity, a pillar of trade, and a healing elixir around the world.

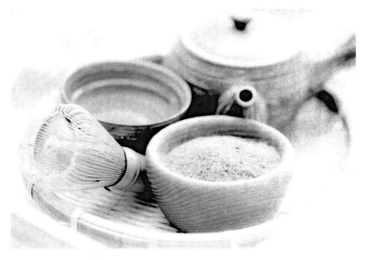

Enter Matcha

There are thousands of varieties of tea. Just as many teas are out there, there are an equal or greater number of ways to consume it.

Few people know that the current practice of drinking powdered tea in the Japanese tea ceremony is actually from the Song Dynasty in China. It dates back to over 1,000 years ago. This practice was carried on in Japan, where it is now considered a pillar of Japanese culture. Today, once again, high quality Matcha is being made in China. This tea has a slightly different character than its Japanese counterpart. Both teas have a deep green color and a thick, savory taste and texture. Both are high in EECG[2] and antioxidants. However, Chinese Matcha is smoother, without the bitterness, and it has a rich, smooth, and fresh taste unlike any other.

Radiation and Japan

When the Fukashima plant had the possibility of a reactor melting, down we all sat on edge watching the news and wondering what the outcome would be. We all began to wonder as   well what would happen if this had occurred in our area and if there was a chance of massive contamination. Even as recently as a few weeks from the editing of this book, pieces of debris were still making their way across the Pacific towards the waters of Hawaii and Southern California. Entire houses and pieces of debris were being dragged by the lulling waves of the Pacific into the waterways, jet stream, and other ecosystems of the Pacific Northwest. And with those soothing waves came another more long-term effect of the storm—radiation.

Aside from Zombie Apocalypse movies, the effects of radiation are nothing to laugh at and can have long-term side effects that can last up to 30 years. There is no way to know how far the contamination from the radiation can travel either as all of these aspects completely depend on the waves, wind, and soil and how far it travels from Japan. Radiation seeps into the soil and then makes the greens such as grass, which the cows consume, contaminated. The long-term effects of the radiation will be seen in the soil, the

---

2 *Matcha Tea: For Renowned Cancer Fighting Catechin EGCG Found Only In Green Tea*, http://www.matchasource.com/matcha-health-s/57.htm Retrieved 2.27.2013

fruits, the vegetables, and in the meat supply for many years to come.

The long-term effects of radiation in doses of the Fukashima plant are unknown at the moment. The small effects can be as little as damage to the DNA or as great as multiple generations of deformity. Over the years, we have seen the long-term effects of nuclear disasters such as Nagasaki and Hiroshima, in which the effects have been generationally altering. Still, to this day, the damage of the reproductive organs has caused deformity and other health issues that are unique to that level of radiation. The lack of knowledge of the widespread nature of the radiation in Japan creates a wild card for the consumption of foods grown in the soil.

Decisively, with the negative effects of radiation, unless you have a radiation detector, it is impossible to know if food has been affected. And if the food has had the addition of radiation, there is not a way to tell that the food has been affected without a detector. There are no visible signs of contamination on the outside of the food or in its appearance. Some experts are now saying it is much easier to steer clear of tea and foods from Japan at the moment until the long-term effects of contamination are determined as well as the level of contamination. For the purposes of this book and for this specific reason, we only recommend Chinese origin Matcha teas.

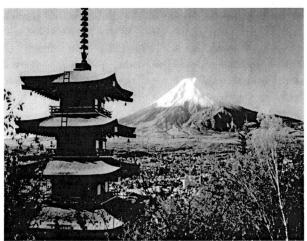

Chapter 2: History of Matcha

Tea is the second most consumed beverage in the world after water itself. Chinese legend heralds that tea was accidentally discovered more than 5,000 years ago when Shennong, a noble farmer in China, had a few tea leaves swept from a nearby growing bush into an open air kettle where water was being boiled. He noticed an instant change in the flavor and properties of the water and sampled it for himself. He then recognized that the drink had a refined taste and decided he would go to the emperor and present the new drink as a cure for health issues. Shennong did not know that he was, in fact, starting a health trend that would not just put him in the good graces of the emperor but would start a new way in which man consumed beverages.

The emperor heralded tea as a gift from the gods and began a regular cultivation of it in China. In the 15th century the art of tea making spread into Japan and was cultivated by the Zen monks that were traveling back and forth across the borders of China and Japan. Within their monasteries, they began the cultivation of green tea and specifically of Matcha. The tea was known to spread clarity to mental faculties and to calm the burdened spirit of the drinker.

Matcha became the staple of the Japanese tea ceremony for years and an art form that women of the upper class as well as Geishas (entertainers) would learn for the many powerful businessmen that they would entertain. They would learn to pass relief and stimulation in the form of the elaborate ritual that would continue to invigorate and expand the properties of the mind.

Kinds of Tea

Teas are much like wines in the aspect that they take on their environment. There is a certain local connection with teas that cannot be denied. Tea picks up aspects of wind, environment, taste, and color based on the soil it is grown in and the characteristics of the region. For this reason, some teas are more robust and spicy than others and teas are as defining as they are unique in their kinds. There are, in fact, nine different kinds of tea:

White Tea: This tea has a sweeter aroma and a warmer smell. These leaves are picked very early and are very tender they are very high in antioxidants. The taste is sweet, slightly malty and not bitter at all.

Green Tea: Green tea has a slightly stronger taste to other kinds of tea as it is never oxidized. It is fresh, green, vegetal, and grassy. Many green teas have had a flavor added to them so that they are actually a little less harsh. It is often possible to get different kinds of tea that are infused with lemon, raspberry, or other flavors.

Oolong Tea: This has a spicy aroma and is ruddy in color. These have lower caffeine content than many of the other teas and for this reason are sweet and fragrant. They tend to move in flavor from spicy all the way to caramel like.

Black Tea: Black tea is the most common form of tea in the U.S. and Europe. It has a slightly stronger taste and a warmer smell. For this reason, the tea is often consumed with milk and sugar or lemon. The taste and smells of black tea can be as varied as the fragrant English Breakfast and move all the way to the more acidic kinds like James Earl Gray.

Herbal Teas: Herbal teas, in fact, are not teas; these are called tisanes. Typically caffeine free, they are usually an infusion of plants and other items. The tastes and smells of the teas can be as varied as the different kinds of ingredients that are used in their production. For this reason, these teas are low in calories and varied in tastes.

Rooibos Teas: These teas are made from a blooming bush in South Africa and are poured over ice or enjoyed hot. They are referred to as Red Tea and have a very fragrant smell and an almost candied taste without the addition of sugar or milk.

Mate Tea: This is made from the leaves and stem of the Yerba plant and taste very similar to coffee. It has a very earthy smell when enjoyed in the traditional way as well and is very pungent. It also has a very acidic quality similar to green tea when tasted, and is sometimes called bitter to an untrained palate.

Blooming Teas: These are handcrafted with elements of flowers put into them. These teas allow the user to drink and enjoy and have the experience of watching them open during the consumption. These teas are usually given to a love or significant other. These teas have the fragrant smell of the flowers used to create them. Also, the taste is slightly weak as it is made with a flower in it and mostly tea. The taste is light and slightly grassy and is not pungent but rather has a sweet smell.

Tea Blends: These teas include an exotic mix of any of the teas listed above with other options. For example, you could mix peppermint and chai to get the taste of your exact specifications. The smell and the taste of the tea are completely different depending on the fusion of the teas.

Matcha and the Japanese Tea Ritual

After becoming Japan's favorite tea, Matcha was part of the elaborate tea ceremony that began in the 12th century. The way of tea became a highly ornamental and distinctive process that included the tea being allowed to dry out in the sun for 30 days prior to picking it. The tea drying in this manner increased the chlorophyll in the tea, which added a richer and more robust green color and taste, which was distinctly that of Matcha.

In Japan, the ceremony was so prized that it would be performed whether in a home, a tea room, a presentation house, or outdoors. The hand motions of the ceremony were also very practiced and could take many hours and days to master for the young lady who was going to be performing the ritual.

At the beginning of the ritual, in front of the guest, the host will clean the tea pot, bowls, and the tea scoop. Following this cleaning, the tea powder is then added into the bowl of the guest, and it is topped with piping hot water. After it is topped with hot water, the Matcha and hot water are whisked together, forming a tea paste. Then, water is added to the bowl of the guest, again, to thin the mixture. Following this step, the host initiates a bow as the guest then picks up the bowl and sips from it. If there are multiple guests, the bowl will be passed among them until it returns to the host. Then, the host will begin the steps over again.

Tea, and the serving of it, has taken on an art status in some forms in Japan as there are tea rooms that charge up to a $2,800.00 sitting fee. There are also teas and derivations of Matcha in China that have added exotic ingredients costing a reported $155.00 per ounce. The tea room business is a full-time business in and of itself in Paris, London, Delhi, Tokyo, and Shanghai. The tea ceremonies, as well as Matcha, have become staples of the Western and Eastern economies.

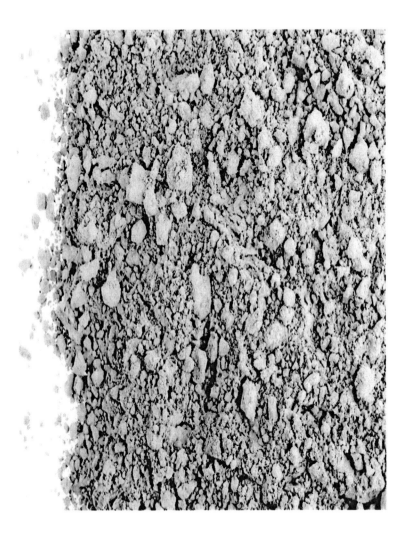

Chapter 3: Sun Tanning and Shaved Mice: An Amazing Experiment

Sun-Tanning, Shaved Mice, and DNA Repair: The Miracle of Green Tea

"The DNA repair ability of a cell is vital to the integrity of its genome and thus to its normal functioning and that of the organism. Many genes that were initially shown to influence life span have turned out to be involved in DNA damage repair and protection. "The genetics of human longevity" Warren S. Browner, MD.

After getting a generous sun-tan treatment, nearly a dozen small, shaved mice scurry across a brightly lit laboratory table. No, the mice are not part of some cruel test of a new sun tan lotion. Rather, they are the subject of Doctor SK Katiyar's latest published study on green tea and its potential to repair DNA.

Doctor Katiyar is one of the University of Alabama's brightest scientists. Doctor Katiyar, along with his cohorts at the National Institute of Public Health and the Environment in the Netherlands, are simultaneously conducting a study to see if green tea may have any potential to promote a better environment to repair DNA within an organism.

The mice have been fed water that contained a type of antioxidant found in green tea (polyphenols) for at least one week before exposing them to UV radiation. The control group of mice was fed drinking water without green tea polyphenols.

Like many humans that are exposed to potentially harmful sunlight, all the mice have been exposed to damaging UV radiation. If Doctor Katiyar's assumption is correct, their DNA would normally be damaged from the UV light.

Under a microscope, the mice are examined, their skin is biopsied and analyzed, their DNA checked, and their immune responses tested. Doctor Katiyar lifts his eyeglasses and smiles. This time something is very different.

Compared with the control group, the mice treated with green tea polyphenols had reduced immunosuppression from the UV radiation. This means that their immune systems were far stronger than the control group's immune systems in battling the harmful effects of the UV radiation.

According to Warren S. Browner. MD in his published "The genetics of human longevity," the DNA repair ability of a cell is vital to the integrity of its genome and thus to its normal functioning and that of the organism. Many genes that were initially shown to influence life span have turned out to be involved in DNA damage repair and protection.[3]

A red light flashes as an indication that the day's experiments are over. Doctor Katiyar sits down at his desk and has a Skype video chat with his counterparts at the National Institute of Public Health and the Environment in the Netherlands.

They have more exciting news. This same group of mice also showed more rapid repair of DNA damaged by UV radiation. Further, the study showed that green tea polyphenols increased the levels of some nucleotide excision repair genes, which allow for DNA repair, and showed more rapid repair of DNA damaged by UV radiation.

The scientists sip a hot cup of their favorite MatchaDNA green tea drink as they smile and toast their accomplishments. Today was a good day.

---

3 (http://nccam.nih.gov/research/results/spotlight/022110.htm) in the journal Cancer Prevention Research, the details of the story have been dramatized by me. I was not present at the study and the story is solely my impression of how it could have happened.

Green Tea Extract Protects Against Brain Damage in Rodent HIV

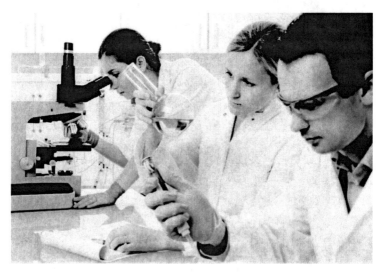

In Tampa in 2007 an amazing study took place. This involved a compound from green tea that diminished the brain toxicity of proteins from HIV. There is a disorder called AIDS dementia that is now one of the most complicated and non-treatable aspects of AIDS. However, with the Florida discovery, a new treatment may be possible.

Brian Giunta MD led a study at the University of Florida; in 2007 he shared with the world his amazing study results. His study was based on a new mouse model of HIV-related dementia. The outcome suggests that EGCG, a component derived from Matcha, may be a natural treatment for HIV-related dementia. Many of the current treatments, when used in conjunction with green tea extract, may prove to penetrate deeper into the cerebral cortex than other more traditional treatments alone.

The aspects of dementia are some of the most complicated aspects of HIV, which begins with the deterioration of the brain and starts with short-term memory loss and leads to the deterioration of complex thinking and, finally, motor skills.

HIV dementia is caused by the direct effects of HIV on the brain through the secretion of toxins, which cause debilitating effects on the brain's neutrons. Giunta found that mice with doses of HIV proteins Gp120 and Tat with cytokine developed brain damage. Giunta then used EGCG and treated the mice with the extract. By doing this, the mice saw their neurotoxicity overcome and also showed the same results in cell studies and in the mouse model of the disease.[4]

Giunta proceeded in his study by harvesting neurons from the mice and then exposing them to the HIV influences. Following this, he added EGCG to the mix and noticed that the green tea kept the cytokine from preventing the death and damage of the neurons. The tea also kept the damage from occurring in live mice as well.

---

[4] green tea extract protects against brain damage in new mouse model of hiv-related dementia. (05, 2007 01). Retrieved from
http://hscweb3.hsc.usf.edu/health/now/?p=129

Chapter 4: The Science Background of Matcha

Research on the science of tea began not in Japan or China but in India. In 1891 a joint committee of the Indian Tea Association and the Agricultural Association of Bengal came together, establishing the first laboratory in which tea could be investigated for its healing properties. After seeing it prescribed by doctors and other wise men, both Eastern and Western societies decided to put the research to the test. Following this, well over one hundred years of research with tea ensued. And of these different studies, some of the most extensive have come from the U.S. by the American Cancer Association while hailing tea as the catch all cure for many ailments. It appears, after all the research and time investment, that the early medical specialists may have been, in fact, correct.

Tea became a formally researched phenomenon in Japan in 1993 with the founding of the formal Tea Research Institute. (Although this organization had operated in a different incarnation since 1957.) Research began to determine what the restorative properties of tea were and why it was so potent. So interested was the crowd that a movement towards a professional master's degree in tea began, and thus was born the discipline of tea study. It has become a full-time profession in the East, with scholars coming to the institute from 37 different international countries, including France, the U.K., and the U.S.[5]

In the U.S., serious tea research and its restorative properties began in 1994 with the study of cancer. Researchers were curious to see if all the results coming out of the East with the changes in the patients through the influence of tea could be reproduced in the West. Trials began specifically with green tea as it was rumored to be the most potent and the most effective of all of the teas.[6]

In order to understand a whole, as Aristotle determined, first you must understand the sum of its parts. What is it about green tea, and specifically Matcha, that had the scientists so amazed? Here

---

[5] *The Tea Institute*, http://www.teausa.com/ 2.27.2013
[6] FDA.govhttp://www.fda.gov/aboutfda/whatwedo/history/milestones/ucm128305.htm Retrieved 2.26.2013

are some of the properties of Matcha that were being examined. We will spend time later discussing the results in the lab.

Properties of Matcha

Of all of the green teas that the institutes have hailed, the best by far is Matcha. Matcha is the only tea that is consumed in the full leaf. For this reason, it is much easier to absorb all of the nutrients and vitamins. Matcha is shaded before it is prepared so that it has a natural green color; this is because the tea has begun to produce more chlorophyll in the shade. The addition of more chlorophyll gives it more nutrients; the darker the color of the tea, the stronger the taste the tea will have. For example, those with a dark, almost forest green color will have a very vegetable-like taste to them, while those teas which are much lighter in color will have a less vegetable-like taste but rather a more tea-like taste. Matcha is also picked by hand so that the best and freshest leaves are chosen without being mechanically processed without discrimination. Being handpicked, the pickers choose simply the best and leave the rest of the leaves.

Matcha, before being powdered, is called "tencha" after it is picked. It is placed under reed mats for two to three weeks and is dried. Following the drying, the tea is then ground into the fine powder that makes up the basis of Matcha. There are, to date, nine different kinds of green tea on the market that have become the obsession of the scientific community for their holistic and restorative properties. And yet, of all of the teas that have been studied, one and only one has remained the darling of the community. That is Matcha. For all of its healing properties, the tea has remained the uncontested winner for healing, mental stasis, clear thinking, well-being, and long-term benefits. Next, we will discuss exactly what these benefits are in more detail as we delve into the labs of the scientists and see what the take away of this amazing tradition has, in fact, become.

The Essence of Matcha

Catechins: These are the elements of tea that add a huge amount of antioxidants into the mix. These decrease oxidization in the body and help with the destruction of free radicals. By decreasing the damage of free radicals, the body is able to use the antioxidants to fight cancer, aging, high blood pressure, and other health issues.[7]

Caffeine: It gets a bad reputation as it causes jitters if over consumed. However, caffeine is actually quite healthy in small doses as it can lower carcinogens, stimulates the heart and the cardiovascular system, and also acts as a diuretic in the system. Caffeine actually contains antioxidants and assists the body with alertness and mental clarity in moderation. For this reason overconsumption can cause an issue, but provided that the user exercises caution, there is also the ability to stimulate the nervous and serotonin production.

Fluoride (naturally occurring): If you do not drink tap water, this is something that is poorly missing in bottled water. Despite the anti-fluoride conspiracy theorists the clinical efficacy of fluoride has been repeatedly proven. Fluoride assists the body with preventing tooth decay and strengthening the enamel for a white and clean smile.[8]

Vitamin B: There are many kinds of Vitamin B. It stimulates the nervous system, and it also assists the body with breaking down protein. It aids in the repair of nerve and skin cells and helps the body with maintaining the brain and spinal cord repair. Vitamin B also assists with the repair of cellular function and assists in the maintenance of the cholesterol in the body.[9]

Vitamin C: This lovely vitamin assists with fighting colds as well as in lowering the stress in the body. Vitamin C also assists in the production of collagen and the youthfulness of the skin. Vitamin C helps the body in the repair of damaged cells and the prevention of free radicals.

Vitamin E: This vitamin assists with sun damage following a burn, and it aids as well in the damage done to the body by free radicals.

---

[7] *The Health Benefits of Matcha*: http:// http://www.sharecare.com/question/how-matcha-green-tea-boost-metabolism. Retrieved 2.26.2013
[8] *Lipophilic and Hydrophilic Antioxidant Capacities of Common Foods in the United States, Journal of Agricultural Food Chemistry* 2004, 52, 4026-4037 // ORAC Analysis on Matcha Green Tea: Brunswick Laboratories Retrieved 2.26.2013
The analysis is based on Kiseki Matcha Organic Chado
[9] *Caffeine Is Not Bad When Consumed In Moderation:*
http://www.topendsports.com/health/caffeine.htm Retrieved 2.16.2013

Vitamin E also assists the body in the production of cellular energy and in the transportation of energy throughout the body.[10]

GABA: This assists with neurotransmission of information, thoughts, and synaptual information in the brain. Also, it assists with the control of the blood pressure in the cardiovascular system by sending regulating pulses from the brain.[11] Theanine also plays a role in the formation of gamma amino butrylic acid (GABA), which may further contribute to the relaxing effects of theanine-containing products, such as Matcha powder and brewed green tea. GABA is a neurotransmitter that has been shown to influence the release of the neurotransmitters dopamine and serotonin.

Flavonoids: Because of their antioxidant qualities, they assist in strengthening the walls of the red blood cells and also help in decreasing swelling and inflammation in other parts of the body.[12] Flavonoids are in tea and are a protein derivative produced by chlorophyll, which assists in inflammation and in bone health.

Theanine: As a naturally occurring amino acid in tea, it assists in the transmission of information and also helps the natural sleep cycle. Like Melatonin, Theanine has a unique combination of acids and proteins that aid the body in staying alert during the appropriate times as well as helping the body regulate time for the sleeping cycle. It is also a natural mood enhancer as it attributes to a sense of well-being and restfulness.[13]

---

[10] *Green Tea and Fluoride:* http://blog.teavana.com/post/2008/07/10/Green-Tea-and-Fluoride.aspx Retrieved 2.26.2013
[11] *Discover Matcha Tea:* http://www.drweil.com/drw/u/ART02050/Matcha-Tea.html Andrew Weil Retrieved 2.26.2013
[12] *Discover Matcha Tea:* http://www.drweil.com/drw/u/ART02050/Matcha-Tea.html Andrew Weil Retrieved 2.26.2013
[13]. Mason (2001) April 7 (2): 91-95 Alternative and Complementary Therapies, *200 mg of Zen; L-Theanine Boosts Alpha Waves, Promotes Alert Relaxation*

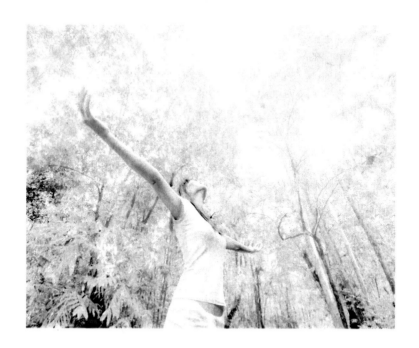

Chapter 5: The Health Benefits of Matcha

So, now we know the history of the drink, the properties, and the ceremony of the tea, which are all well and good. However, the lingering question is: What is it about Matcha that makes it so relevant and makes it stand the test of time? Obviously, it is touted by scientists for its restorative and elixir-like qualities. Do the long-term effects of these results change over time and person to person, or is it merely duplicative on lab rats and not on human beings?

Many studies leave the audience scratching their heads because we find that the studies were conducted on animals but have not been conducted on humans and, of course, the individual chemistry makeup of each person comes into play. Just because something will work for me does not mean it will work for you. What are the qualities that make Matcha a favorable choice for every person?

It is not very often that something is introduced into a culture with as much history as Matcha—stemming back to Chinese royalty and Japanese Zen monks. Obviously, there are facts that commend the tea, not just as a proponent to healthfulness, but also regarding its amazing historical background.

What are the health benefits of Matcha?

Aids in Digestion: The tannins that are in Matcha help with digestion. It is a wonderful cure for people that have constipation or indigestion. The tannins stimulate the activity of the intestinal track and speed up food production in the bowels.[14]

Refreshes Body and Mind: The amount of caffeine that is in Matcha is actually higher than the amount in a cup of coffee; however, it does not give the drinker jitters because of the other ingredients in the tea that aid in the absorption. When it was first developed, it was utilized as a help for staying awake by the royalty in China and Japan. The mind feels more refreshed and active with the infusion of

---

[14] Hara, Yukihiko. Green tea: health benefits and applications. Vol. 106. CRC, 2001.

the caffeine, and this leads to more focused concentration and thought.[15]

Prevents Illness: Matcha contains an extremely high amount of antioxidants and vitamins and assists in preventing most communicable illnesses when it is consumed on a regular basis. The tea contains more antioxidants and differing vitamins than any other tea on the market as it is chocked full of Vitamin B, Vitamin C, Vitamin E, and many other antioxidants and peptides.[16]

Promotes Healthy Skin Tone: Vitamin C aids the body in the production of collagen. Collagen is the same substance that is injected into the face and other areas to reduce lines and wrinkles. Also, Vitamin C creates a healthy glow that gives the sign of youth and vitality as it also helps to even out the skin tone and facilitate healing if there has been a burn or a scar.[17]

Aids in Weight Loss: Many over the counter diet aids in the past few years have resulted from the research that was done on Matcha and other green teas. The extract from Matcha is considered to be the most potent because of the chlorophyll content in the plant and also because of the stimulation that occurs to the metabolism of the subject. Because of the increase in metabolism, people who add Matcha to diet plans with regular exercise typically lose two pounds per week.[18]

Source of Zinc: If you have a zinc deficiency, you might not notice it. Lack of zinc can cause many issues, such as diarrhea, hair loss, acne, issues with the immune system, impotence, skin lesions, slow healing wounds, and slow growth. Zinc plays a crucial role in the body's ability to fight infections, its ability to heal, and in its ability to process nutrients. People who drink alcohol, breastfeeding mothers, people with irritable bowels, and vegetarians are all at risk of developing a zinc deficiency. However, Matcha is an amazing source of zinc and contains a daily supplement if two cups of tea are consumed.[19]

Inhibits Carcinogens: Doctors encourage cancer patients to consume Matcha for the properties of Catechins, which actually are able to

---

[15] Ibid.
[16] Ibid.
[17] Ibid.
[18] Ibid.
[19] Ibid.

suppress the growth of cancer tumors with their slowing and healing properties. In addition to these properties, the antioxidants that are in the tea also have the ability to prevent the damage that carcinogens do to the system. What is a carcinogen, you are asking yourself? It is essentially anything that causes cancer. And these days, that is almost anything. For example, some of these are: fried foods, too much alcohol, and stress. For this reason, carcinogen prevention is much more important than it has been in the past. As our lives get faster and faster and the world gets smaller and smaller, taking that daily pause to supplement your health and increase your sense of well-being will become more and more important. Taking a moment to enjoy that cup of Matcha may be a matter of an opportunity for a decreased incidence of cancer, with cancer having now officially taken its spot among the top ten and as the second most possible cause of death for American consumers.[20]

Lowers Cholesterol Levels: Matcha is able to prevent the hardening of the arteries and the forming of blood clots by utilizing Catechins to move waste throughout the system at a rapid rate. Matcha is becoming a part of the prescription of doctors and nurses alike in an effort to reduce the high levels of issues related to high cholesterol.[21]

Lowers High Blood Pressure: With the spinning pace of life these days, it is amazing just how many people have issues with high blood pressure. Matcha may be a solution for high blood pressure since, when consumed on a daily basis, blood pressure falls significantly in people with the condition. Catechins inhibit the body from being able to allow a rise in blood pressure, which greatly helps the general feeling and stasis of an individual.[22]

The health benefits of Matcha are undeniable as outlined here in this chapter. You really have to ask yourself: In a highly processed diet, how much zinc, Vitamins A, B, D, and C are you consuming? Chances are, by far not enough, and Matcha may be the thing you are missing from your diet. When you look at all of the benefits that Matcha imparts, how many of them are on your list? Are there five to seven, maybe more? In this world of ours, there has never been a greater need for the healing properties that we so ardently desire and

---

[20] Ibid.
[21] Ibid.
[22] Ibid.

demand. Instead of in a new technology, we find those properties here in a five thousand year old tradition.

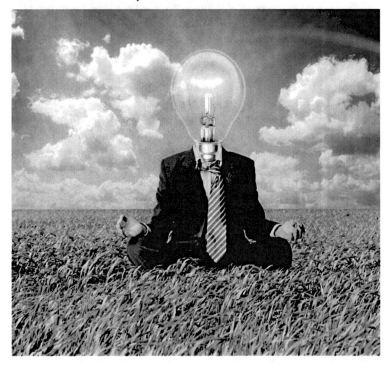

Chapter 6: Clinical Trials on Green Tea and Matcha

In the Journal of Medicinal Food 2009, tests on rats with type 2 diabetes proved that the Matcha tea decreased levels of cholesterol, body sugar, and harmful body fats. The tea also appeared to protect the rats from liver and kidney damage. The Matcha may contain higher levels of antioxidants than other forms of green tea, therefore offering many more health benefits.[23]

There is also some evidence that green tea can help to prevent several forms of cancer. In a review in 2009, scientists decided that the consumption of green tea might reduce the risk of lung cancer, prostate cancer, pancreatic cancer, and colorectal cancer. It is thought to help by fighting off free radicals that damage DNA. It also has been touted as a weight loss product. A study in the *American Journal of Clinical Nutrition* claims that Matcha green tea produces a significant increase in energy expenditure so that it increases thermogenesis (the body's own rate of burning calories) from a normal 8–10% to a 35–43% of daily energy expenditure. With this, no one in the tests noticed any side effects, unlike ephedra, which can raise heart rates and blood pressure.

Middle aged women in groups of 75,000 or more were studied and asked about their green tea consumption. It was found that of these women over 80 percent were consuming tea over three times a week for six weeks. The end result was that there was a 17% reduced rate of GI cancers provided that the person in question was drinking tea at least 3 times a week for 6 weeks.

In 2012, at the University of Strathclyde, a team of researchers made 40 percent of the cancer cells disappear in a patient with a powdered form of Matcha. In the past, these kinds of systems have failed to deliver the result of shrinking the tumors on contact because the concentrate of green tea would have been diluted to an amount that could not be effective. The method of delivery was

---

[23] S. Nechuta, X.-O. Shu, H.-L. Li, G. Yang, B.-T. Ji, Y.-B. Xiang, H. Cai, W.-H. Chow, Y.-T. Gao, W. Zheng. **Prospective cohort study of tea consumption and risk of digestive system cancers: results from the Shanghai Women's Health Study**. *American Journal of Clinical Nutrition*, 2012; 96 (5): 1056 DOI: 10.3945/ajcn.111.031419

modified this time to ensure effective delivery of the compounds by sending the powdered tea mix directly across the cell barrier so it could deliver the maximum amount of potency.[24]

The University of Strathclyde was amazed at their results demonstrated that Matcha is now a possible way to shrink skin cancer and that regular consumption of it could actually prevent skin cancer. [25]

In 2009 there was study led by Columbia University in which men with prostate cancer and women with breast cancer were given powdered Matcha extract. In the women and in the men, the dosage was in powdered caplets of 24 cups per day. For the first 30 days, both women and men experienced a significant amount of shrinking in the tumors they both had. Following this, there was a reduction in the shrinking of the tumors, which Columbia attributed as patients forgetting to keep up with the amount of pills to keep the shrinking going. However, these results were, in fact, very compelling to the community and left them with a hunger to come back with more studies.[26]

Matcha has also been linked to studies of overall improvement in the functioning of the brain; in September of 2012 the Third Medical Military College in China found that the functioning of the brain was greatly stimulated by a chemical in the tea called ECGC, a common antioxidant. The regular consumption by patients of three cups of Matcha a day found that the levels of the antioxidant speeded up the delivery of messages in the brain and the function of memory. In addition to this, there was significant evidence to show that those who consumed the tea also were able to see an increase in the regeneration and the protection of brain cells.

Researchers from Swiss and Basel Universities recently worked in tandem with one another on an interesting study in which they gave their subjects a soft drink that contained Matcha. The soft

---

[24] Antitumor activity of the tea polyphenol epigallocatechin-3-gallate encapsulated in targeted vesicles after intravenous administration. University of Strathclyde, 2012, http://www.ncbi.nlm.nih.gov/pubmed/22891867
[25] Antitumor activity of the tea polyphenol epigallocatechin-3-gallate encapsulated in targeted vesicles after intravenous administration. University of Strathclyde, 2012, http://www.ncbi.nlm.nih.gov/pubmed/22891867
[26] Antitumor activity of the tea polyphenol epigallocatechin-3-gallate encapsulated in targeted vesicles after intravenous administration. University of Strathclyde, 2012, http://www.ncbi.nlm.nih.gov/pubmed/22891867

drink was then given to the subject two times per day. There were 12 men who were given the drink and then were given brain scans. It was found that in the men who consumed the soft drink, the activity in the frontal cortex was stimulated and that the brain, again, began to increase the level of brain cell production (as that of a child). Again, they also witnessed a better memory, quicker retrieval, and faster synapses when being tested on brain memory and testing machines. The differences in the subjects were purportedly so significant that the men vowed they would continue drinking the soft drink, which contained less than a quarter of the green tea antioxidants than found in one glass of Matcha.[27]

Matcha has now been linked to preventing Alzheimer's in a recent study that was conducted by the University of Leeds in which patients with the disease were served green tea supplements four times per day. Alzheimer's occurs when clumps in the brain cells result in memory loss and other issues. It is more difficult for the messages of the brain to be transmitted through the walls and other layers of debris once the disease begins. Matcha infusion into the system is now being shown to break up the existing knots and to help in preventing new ones from forming from the high concentration of antibiotics that are present in the tea. According to the University of Leeds, this study is convincing doctors that the next step for treatment in the field of Alzheimer's may be an entirely new line of drugs which are, in fact, focused on the makeup of Matcha. The higher the level of progression of the Alzheimer's in a patient, the higher the concentration of the portion of Matcha would be in order to increase the net effect of the medicine.[28]

With the aging of the Baby Boomer generation, doctors are racing to attempt to find a sustainable cure for Alzheimer's and for many other memory loss diseases that are beginning to plague over half a million people in Britain and even larger numbers in the U.S. This research conducted by the University of Leeds may, in fact, lead to a new line of drugs.

In addition to the potential benefits seen in the curative properties of Matcha in relation to Alzheimer's, in 2012 in China, as

---

[27] Wiley. "Brainy beverage: Study reveals how green tea boosts brain cell production to aid memory." *ScienceDaily*, 5 Sep. 2012. Web. 27 Feb. 2013.

[28] Wiley. "Brainy beverage: Study reveals how green tea boosts brain cell production to aid memory." *ScienceDaily*, 5 Sep. 2012. Web. 27 Feb. 2013.

a joint effort by China and Japan, a study was conducted on the way that Matcha is able to also assist with glaucoma and with gum disease. [29]

In a study published in *Molecular Nutrition & Food Research*, a team of Chinese researchers discovered that an organic chemical found in green tea, epigallocatechin-3 gallate or EGCG, could improve memory and spatial learning by boosting the generation of brain cells—a process known as neurogenesis.

The compound EGCG is already known for its antioxidant tendencies. But in the Chinese study, EGCG was also shown to be beneficial against age-related degenerative diseases with particular impact on the hippocampus, the part of the brain that processes information from short-term to long-term memory.

For their study, researchers ran tests on two groups of mice, one of which was fed EGCG, and the other acting as a control group. The mice were then trained for several days to find a visible and an invisible platform within a maze.

What researchers found was that the mice treated with the Matcha tea compound required less time to find the hidden platform compared to their counterparts, showing that EGCG can enhance learning and memory by improving object recognition and spatial memory. In the same study, mice with glaucoma, which causes issues with vision and eventual blindness, were also treated with the Matcha extract. The mice were then tested in two groups: one as a control and the other to see the effects on the Matcha mice. The mice had a significant decrease in the severity of their glaucoma as the Matcha assisted by breaking up the fatty deposits that were causing the glaucoma.[30]

Thus far we have seen that Matcha may greatly reduce issues with Alzheimer's, cancer, glaucoma, and also with gum disease. But we are also about to see that recent clinical studies are beginning to

---

[29]. Wiley. "Brainy beverage: Study reveals how green tea boosts brain cell production to aid memory." *ScienceDaily*, 5 Sep. 2012. Web. 27 Feb. 2013.
[30] *Green Tea May Prevent and Heal Eye Ailments Including Glaucoma:*
http://www.machomatcha.com/research/green-tea-may-prevent-andheal-eye-ailments-including-glaucoma 2012

point to lowering blood pressure, lowering cholesterol, and assisting with weight issues.[31]

In October of 2008 Mary Nantz compiled a list of 52 women and 72 men around the age of 29 and gave them a Matcha tea supplement for four weeks. During that time, these patients were measured daily for LDL as well as for blood pressure. It was found that these subjects had between an 8 and 42 percent drop in blood pressure at the conclusion of four weeks, while the LDL levels of the patients also fell between 8 and 12 points. For this reason, she was able to conclude that consuming Matcha will, in fact, lower all of these bad numbers and increase the production of good cholesterol.[32]

With heart disease, and specifically heart attack and stroke, being linked to high blood pressure, scientists are seeking for ways to lower the blood pressure and the cholesterol of their patients in natural ways, without the synthesis of more drugs and other items, which might have long-term side effects. Many of the current drugs that are on the shelves are known to cause longer term and more pressing issues, such as kidney failure. For this reason, as younger and younger people develop issues of blood pressure, it is necessary to find another cure for the issue other than lifetime medication, as this could very likely lead to kidney failure.

All of the natural steps that we are able to take as consumers to assist and to facilitate with our own health greatly lower the cost of health care in the long term and assists with our overall care. As the costs of health care continue to climb and employers are contributing less and less to pensions and healthcare costs, it becomes more the focus of the consumer to ensure that they are doing all they can to decrease the long-term side effects of medicines by finding natural solutions like Matcha.[33]

In another test, in Taiwan in 2004, regarding blood pressure, all of the drinkers of tea that consumed at least half a cup of green tea

[31] *Green Tea May Prevent and Heal Eye Ailments Including Glaucoma:* http://www.machomatcha.com/research/green-tea-may-prevent-andheal-eye-ailments-including-glaucoma 2012

[32]. *Green Tea May Prevent and Heal Eye Ailments Including Glaucoma:* http://www.machomatcha.com/research/green-tea-may-prevent-andheal-eye-ailments-including-glaucoma 2012

[33]. Benelli R, Vene R, Bisacchi D, Garbisa S, Albini A: **Anti-invasive effects of green tea polyphenol epigallocatechin-3-galleate (EGCG), a natural inhibitor of metallo and serine proteases.**

on a daily basis experienced a decrease in blood pressure by 50%. An important health responsibility of each person is also a lurking issue for those who are predisposed to conditions like high blood pressure. In some families, there is simply a predisposition to the condition as it is genetic and there is a history of heart disease. The result of 50% was for people who had already developed high blood pressure. For those who had not developed blood pressure but were merely predisposed to it, after drinking half a cup of Matcha for a year, they saw their chances of predisposition falling by 65% as a sustained, long-term effect. Also, those patients who had taken part in the study were, in fact, all educators or people in very high stress jobs describing themselves as classic "Type A" personalities. By consuming the tea, they also reported an overall better feeling of well-being and calmness than they had prior to beginning the consumption.[34]

Matcha and Weight Loss

In a 90-day study in 2009 in China, Fudan University took a group of moderately overweight Chinese subjects from the ages of 18 to 55 and divided them into four groups. Each group was then allocated a different amount of catechins in the supplement they were given, which ranged from 30–120 mg of catechins per person. Each person consumed two cups of tea daily with the amount of Matcha catechins prescribed; they then were measured at day 30, 60, and 90 to see how they were progressing. The subjects were measured in being overweight, circumference, and body mass.

The subjects were not allowed to consume any other caffeine containing beverages during this time period. The average subject showed a 40% decrease in being overweight and mass and overall improvement in mood and fitness. The researchers concluded that more studies needed to be conducted in other subjects and other populations to ensure that the results were the same across cultural influences.[35]

---

[34] Benelli R, Vene R, Bisacchi D, Garbisa S, Albini A: **Anti-invasive effects of green tea polyphenol epigallocatechin-3-galleate (EGCG), a natural inhibitor of metallo and serine proteases.**

[35] *Green Tea Extract Eradicates Cancer Tumors*, Stephen Adams, Telegraph.uk retrieved 2.27.2013 http://www.telegraph.co.uk/health/healthnews/9490733/Green-tea-extract-eradicates-cancer-tumours.html

Another issue that patients often encounter when trying to lose weight is an issue with slow metabolism. With the introduction of foods that have steroids and supplements like estrogen inside of them, aside from the body's natural PH being off slightly, metabolism can be slowed down. Consumption of Matcha is shown to increase the speed of the metabolism and further assist in weight loss and also in the burning of calories.[36]

With any weight loss plan, the subject learns very quickly that they really have two choices. They can, in fact, reduce their calorie intake or increase the amount of calories they are burning. In a recent study, it was determined that subjects that drank Matcha saw an increase in calorie burning. The study was published in *American Journal of Clinical Nutrition* and focused on the question of whether weight loss was due to Matcha or whether it was due to the consumption of the caffeine in a beverage. The group was then divided into two subject groups: one had Matcha and one had caffeine. It was found that the group that had consumed the Matcha raised their metabolism by 40% over a 90-day period while there was no increase in the metabolism of the subjects that had consumed the caffeine. For this reason, it was conclusive for the researchers that, in fact, the effects had come not from the caffeine but from the tea.

Matcha and green tea are now proving themselves as a sunscreen as well. In Germany in 2011, sixty women, for 90 days, consumed a green tea beverage two times a day. Following this period, when the women were subjected to ultraviolet rays, they were found to have a much better resistance to the sun and were even able to see some prevention against burning. For many years as well it has been suggested by health stores to put green tea extract directly on a burn so that the skin is able to soak up the extract, which then is able to aid in relieving the pain, cooling the burn, and allowing healing at a cellular level due to the amount of antioxidants combating the cellular damage that occurs in a burn.[37]

---

[36] *Green Tea Extract Eradicates Cancer Tumors*, Stephen Adams, Telegraph.uk retrieved 2.27.2013 http://www.telegraph.co.uk/health/healthnews/9490733/Green-tea-extract-eradicates-cancer-tumours.html
[37] *Green Tea Extract Eradicates Cancer Tumors*, Stephen Adams, Telegraph.uk retrieved 2.27.2013 http://www.telegraph.co.uk/health/healthnews/9490733/Green-tea-extract-eradicates-cancer-tumours.html

In August of 2012 the University of Strathclyde began looking at the effects of green tea extract on the growth of skin cancer tumors. The results were very surprising. Instead of having the subject drink the tea, it was necessary to inject the subjects with the extract directly into the tumor. They were injected with a part of the extract referred to as EGCG to treat the issue at hand. Tests were done on two types of skin cancer: epidermoid carcinoma, which forms scales on the surface of the skin, and melanoma, which often develops in people who have moles on their skin. In both studies, forty percent of tumors vanished, while thirty percent of tumors in carcinoma cases and twenty percent in melanoma cases shrank. Ten percent of melanoma tumors were stabilized; they did not grow or shrink.[38]

Following all of the information out there proves there is little doubt of the importance of drinking Matcha. The numbers and evidence simply do not lie. Drinking Matcha is a solution that will pay dividends for years to come for better health.

[38]. *Green Tea Extract Eradicates Cancer Tumors*, Stephen Adams, Telegraph.uk retrieved 2.27.2013 http://www.telegraph.co.uk/health/healthnews/9490733/Green-tea-extract-eradicates-cancer-tumours.html

Chapter 7: EGCG—A Revolution in Motion

Epigallocatechin gallate (EGCG) is also known as Gallic acid and is found in green tea and is particularly potent in Matcha. Currently it is one of the most researched aspects of tea research. It is being utilized as a possible solution for several areas of concern to health:

- **HIV:** ECGC is currently being studied as a means to blocking dementia related to HIV. Its implementation is being considered a possible solution to clumps of brain matter by utilizing EGCG in a very concentrated form. [39]

- **Cancer:** EGCG is currently also being used to prevent the spread of brain, prostate, and cervical cancer. EGCG is being used to inhibit the growth and replication of cancer cells. [40]

- **Chronic Fatigue:** ECGC is very effective in assisting with water retention and inflammation and assists in activating the body against Alpha and Beta Proteins. [41]

- **Sjorgren's Syndrome:** ECGC, when consumed on a regular basis, is in fact able to prevent the inception of auto immune diseases. [42]

- **Endometriosis:** The University of Oxford has experimented with inserting implants in the interior female cavity with both Vitamin E and ECGC. It was found that the ECGC was able to

---

[39] Williamson MP, McCormick TG, Nance CL, Shearer WT (December 2006). "Epigallocatechin gallate, the main polyphenol in green tea, binds to the T-cell receptor, CD4: Potential for HIV-1 therapy". *The Journal of Allergy and Clinical Immunology* 118 (6): 1369–74. doi:10.1016/j.jaci.2006.08.016. PMID 17157668
[40] **Shankar S, Ganapathy S, Hingorani SR, Srivastava RK.:** *EGCG inhibits growth, invasion, angiogenesis and metastasis of pancreatic cancer* **Department of Biochemistry, University of Texas Health Science Center at Tyler, Tyler, Texas**
[41] Sachdeva AK, Kuhad A, Chopra K.; *Epigallocatechin gallate ameliorates behavioral and biochemical deficits in rat model of load-induced chronic fatigue syndrome*: University Institute of Pharmaceutical Sciences, UGC Centre of Advanced Study, Panjab University, Chandigarh, India.
[42] Medical College of Georgia. "Green Tea And EGCG May Help Prevent Autoimmune Diseases." *ScienceDaily*. 20 Apr. 2007. Web. 27 Feb. 2013.

aid in the repair of the scar tissue in the endometrium wall. [43] Spinal Muscular Atrophy: ECGC is known to assist the facilitation of cell growth and to help repair cells, muscle, and bone.[44]

- **Neurodegeneration:** ECGC aids in preventing the *brain from deteriorating when significant levels* of green tea are consumed. This has been verified in a recent study by the Journal of Neurochemistry.[45]

- **Cb1 Receptor:** EGCG has been found to assist in inflammation and also in assisting with fat blocking and production. This has been examined by the University of Rosenberg in Germany in great detail and was first published in 2012. [46]

- **Periapical Lesions:** At National Taipei University in Taiwan, an experiment was conducted to see the effects of ECGC on bone loss and lesions. The results were rather staggering as it was concluded that ECGC actually does diminish CCL2 osteoblasts, or lesions, in humans. [47]

---

[43] *Natural therapies assessment for the treatment of endometriosis Hum Reprod (2013) 28(1): 178-188:* Oxford University 2012.
http://humrep.oxfordjournals.org/content/24/3/608.short
[44] *Green Tea Extract Benefits(2013) 28(1): 178-188:* Oxford University 2012.
http://humrep.oxfordjournals.org/content/24/3/608.short
[45] **Yona Levites, *Journal of Neurochemistry Volume 78, Issue 5, pages 1073–1082,* September 2001**
[46] University of Rosenburg: Phytomedicine Volume 17, Issue 1, January 2010, Pages 19–22
[47]. EGCG diminishes CCL2 expression in human osteoblasts National Taiwan University O.H. Shock, 2008.

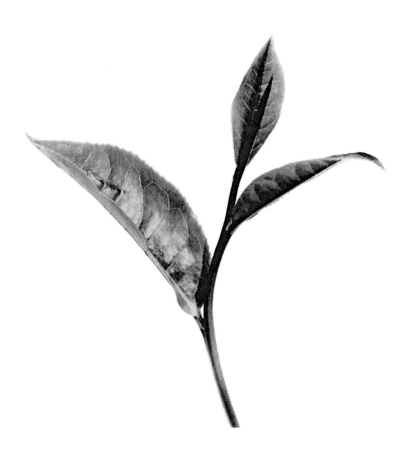

Matcha Green Tea

Chapter 8: Matcha DNA—A Chinese Revolution

Chinese Matcha is smoother, more round in the mouth, and less bitter than its Japanese counterpart. Given the vegetal experience of some Japanese Matcha, it is incorporated into Bubble tea or other recipes instead of being consumed in its original form. As far as the Chinese counterpart goes, it is more easily digested and consumed because of the smoothness of its character and lack of harsh taste.

In addition to this, Chinese Matcha is always harvested by hand as well as there being a different farming technique in China than in Japan. In China, tea is heavily regulated, and much of the gardening and raising of the Matcha is handled organically without the use of pesticides; all is tended by hand.

Currently, with the radiation in the soil in Japan, the long-term effects of consuming produce and products grown in the soil are touch and go at best; to bring everything full circle, we know that it is impossible from looking at the food to tell if there is, in fact, radioactive damage to it. Considering the reasons you are consuming Matcha to begin with, that is not something you want to gamble with when the long-term effects are not known and will not be known for many years to come.

Facts about Matcha

- Ancient, 5,000-year-old tradition that originated in China
- Assisted royalty with ailments
- Hand-picked
- May increase physical energy
- Contains Theanine that may help one's sleep cycle
- May increase metabolism
- May decrease risk of certain cancers
- May help with cell rejuvenation
- May help with beautiful skin
- May lead to greater mental clarity
- Is great to cook with
- May lower cholesterol
- May lower blood pressure[48]

---

[48] Hara, Yukihiko. *Green tea: health benefits and applications.* Vol. 106. CRC, 2001.

Chapter 9: Recipes for Matcha

Matcha Green Tea: Straight Shot

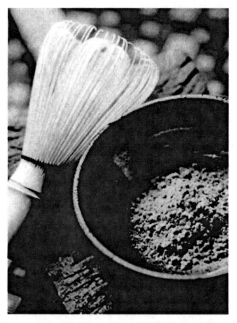

The trick to preparing a ceremonial style Matcha green tea is to preheat the cup or bowl and then to add tea powder and whisk to perfection before adding the remaining water. Never use boiling water. Do use hot water.

- Pre-warm your cup or bowl with hot water.

- Put 1 pouch or 1 tsp (2.5 grams) Matcha into a cup.

- Add 2 ounces of hot water and stir with a whisk or milk frother until well whisked.

- Pour 4-5 oz of hot water into your favorite Matcha bowl or teacup.

- Whisk again to perfection.

- Enjoy quietly.

Making The Ultimate Matcha Latte

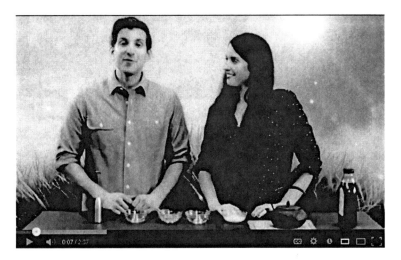

Matcha Latte

Preparation

- Whilst traditional Matcha is served without milk or sweetener, it's common to find a green tea latte in your local Starbucks or other neighborhood café.

- Matcha lattes can be a very satisfying and a supremely delicious alternative to your morning coffee or a warm, sweet after-dinner treat.

- This recipe uses Almond Milk. You may substitute hemp milk, milk, half & half, soy milk, or non-dairy creamer.

Note: Foam will vary due to fat content of the milk and the type of product used.

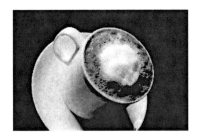

Matcha Green Tea Latte

Prepare cafe style beverages at home.

The trick to preparing a cafe style Matcha green tea latte is to make the tea first, then add the hot milk and foam.

- Pre-warm your cup with hot water.
- Put 1 pouch or 1 tsp (2.5 grams) Matcha into a cup.
- Add 2 ounces of hot water and stir with a whisk or milk frother.
- Pour 4-5 oz steamed* milk into your favorite Matcha bowl or teacup.
- Add milk from frother or froth milk in cup using hand held frother.
- Scoop foamy milk on top.
- Sprinkle with cinnamon, Matcha, or cocoa powder.

Optional

- Add vanilla, almond, or mint flavors.
- Sweeten with stevia, honey, or agave nectar.

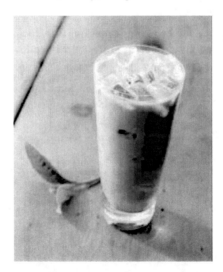

Iced Matcha Green Tea Latte

Blend a chilled Matcha green tea latte using a classic martini shaker.

- Add 2 tsp <u>Matcha</u> into a martini shaker.

- Add 2 oz hot water or milk and stir until Matcha becomes smooth.

- Fill shaker with 1 cup ice.

- Add 6 oz milk – cow, hemp, almond, soy, or rice

- Shake well to blend green tea powder with milk.

- Strain your chilled green tea latte over a tall glass with fresh ice.

Optional

- Froth milk in a Nespresso or Bodum Milk Frother and spoon foam over the top.

- Add flavor with pomegranate juice, coconut water, or lemon grass.

- Add a pinch of Matcha or cinnamon over the top.

- Sip through a straw.

Adjust quantities to your personal taste. We are creating a new tradition here. There are no hard rules. Some people may prefer more milk and more tea or vice versa.

Beyond Green Tea Lattes: Anything Is Possible

In addition to Matcha green tea lattes, you can experiment by adding to yogurt shakes, milk drinks, and cocktails. Use a blender for mixing with ingredients like yogurt and ice cream. Use a hand held milk frother for cafe drinks and a martini shaker for iced-tea cocktails and mocktails.

Aside from just consuming Matcha in the traditional tea manner, many new and exciting recipes have been invented. These recipes allow for you to experience the benefits of Matcha with a new and exciting twist.

Dorayaki with Matcha and Strawberries

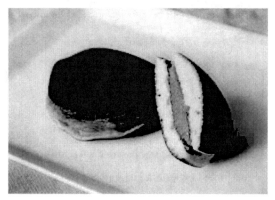

Ingredients:

(For 6 units)

2 eggs	Baking soda 1.5g
Sugar 110g	Water 25ml
Honey 12g	Flour 125g
Mirin (sweet sake) 6g	Soy sauce 2g

Preparation:

1. In a bowl, mix eggs and sugar.

2. Add mirin, honey, and soy sauce, and mix again.

3. Dissolve the baking soda into the water.

4. Add the sifted flour into the egg mixture gradually.

5. Leave the dough about 30 minutes.

6. Heat frying pan or hot plate without adding oil; cook the dough. (We recommend using a Teflon frying pan.)

7. When bubbles begin to form and appear of the surface of the cake, turn the pancake over in the pan.

8. Cook 10 seconds more and cool the pancake.

9. Put Matcha butter cream* and strawberries between the pancake.

Matcha Spongy Cake

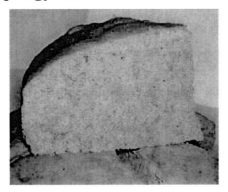

Ingredients:

3 egg yolks
40 g sugar
40g almond powder

Vanilla Essence
3 egg whites
40 g sugar
40 g flour
Matcha green tea powder 8 g
(Matcha Cream)
100 g cream

1 teaspoon of Matcha green tea powder
(Chocolate Cream)
100 g cream
60 g white chocolate
80 g of black chocolate
(Matcha Syrup)
100cc water
20 g sugar
1 teaspoon of Matcha green tea powder

Preparation:

1. Mix egg yolks and sugar. Add almond powder and vanilla essence and mix well.

2. Make a meringue with egg whites and sugar.

3. Add one third of the meringue into the mixture, then add the flour and mix it. Add the remaining meringue and mix again.

4. Bake the mixture in the oven at 200°C (400°F) for 8 minutes.

5. Prepare Matcha cream. Boil the cream and melt chocolate inside. Whip the cream and add Matcha.

6. Prepare chocolate cream in the same way.

7. Prepare Matcha syrup. Heat water; add sugar and Matcha green tea and mix well.

8. Remove the sponge cake from oven and divide into 3 equal parts and moisten them with syrup.

9. **Assemble the cake in the following order**: First of all, place one square of sponge cake on the baking sheet and moisten it gently with Matcha syrup. Next, put on chocolate cream. Next, put another square of sponge cake on. Next, put Matcha cream on the cake. Next, put another square of sponge cake on, etc.

10. Finally, melt black chocolate and put on the cake.

Matcha Sweets

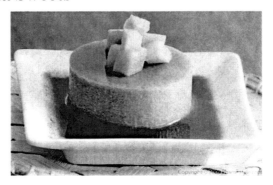

Traditional Japanese snacks are usually healthy because many of the ingredients are natural and the main ingredient is red azuki beans, known as bean paste "anko." Yokan is a popular Japanese sweet made from "anko," often served at tea time. Here is a new recipe of another type of Yokan made from white beans and Japanese green tea Matcha.

1. Soak the agar in water for 15 minutes. Place the agar and water into a pot. Cook under low heat while stirring occasionally with a wooden spatula. Add sugar, and when the mixture is an even consistency, turn off the heat.

250cc of water   30 g of sugar

5 g of agar powder

2. In a bowl mix Matcha powder with water. Add white bean paste (shiro-an) and mix well.

5 g of Matcha   10cc of water

white bean paste (shiro-an) 300g *(recipe will be published soon)

3. Add 2. into 1. After boiling a little, put the mixture in a mold that has been moistened with water. Refrigerate until gelled. Remove mixture from the mold and cut with knife into tiny pieces.

Matcha Tiramisu

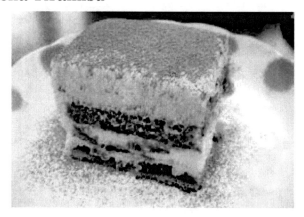

Ingredients:

For mascarpone cream:
65 g mascarpone
1 egg yolk
12 g of sugar
1 teaspoon of rum
100cc of whipped cream
1 tablespoon of Matcha

For white sponge cake:
2 egg yolks
40 g sugar
50cc of milk
40 g flour
2 egg whites

For Matcha sponge cake:
2 egg yolks
40 g sugar
50cc of milk
40 g of flour
2 egg whites
1 tablespoon of Matcha

For decoration:
(First layer)
10 g of powdered sugar
(Second layer)
10 g of Matcha

Preparation:

1. Prepare Matcha sponge cake. In a bowl, mix the egg yolks, sugar, milk, and Matcha previously sifted. Then, add the flour also pre-sifted. In another bowl, prepare meringue, beating egg whites with a mixer. Mix the dough and meringue.

2. In another bowl, prepare white sponge cake. Mix white yolks, sugar, and milk. Add the flour well sifted. In another bowl, prepare meringue, beating egg whites. Mix the dough and meringue.

3. Put 1. & 2. into two square molds respectively. Bake 15 minutes at 180 °C (350°F).

4. Make mascarpone cream mixing egg yolk, sugar and rum. Add Matcha powder. Then, add the whipped cream and mix all lightly.

5. Cut baked sponge cakes in half horizontally. First, put green sponge cake and spread mascarpone cream over cake. Put white cake over and spread cream over cake. Repeat.

6. On the top of the cake, drizzle powdered sugar to totally cover the surface of the cake.

7. Drizzle Matcha powder over cake to totally cover the surface of the cake.

Matcha Jelly

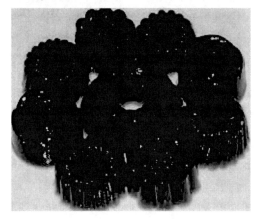

Ingredients:

Matcha powder: 1 Tbsp   Gelatin powder: 10 g

Sugar: 1.5 Tbsp   Whipped cream for topping

Water: 500ml

Preparation:

1. Put Matcha powder, sugar, and 10ml of hot water in a cup and mix well with a spoon.

2. Put gelatin powder in a bowl and add 100ml of water and mix well.

3. Boil 400ml of water.

4. Pour the hot water into the gelatin powder.

5. Add 1. to 4.

6. Pour 5. into serving cups or containers and cool them out of the refrigerator for a while.

7. Cool them in the refrigerator for 2 hours.

8. Top with some whipped cream and sprinkle Matcha on before serving.

Matcha Ciccolata

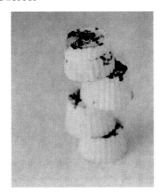

Ingredients:

(2 persons) (Makes 30 small chocolates sized 1.5cm x 1.5cm x 1.5cm)

10ml of cream	150 g of white chocolate
5 g of butter	1 tablespoon dried red fruit (3 g)

1 tablespoon of Matcha to mix with chocolate (3 g)

1 tablespoon of Matcha for sprinkling (3 g)

Preparation:

1. Heat the cream in a small saucepan over medium heat.

2. Crush white chocolate and put it into the cream and melt, stirring.

3. Add 3 g Matcha and stir with a rubber spatula until smooth.

4. Crush berries and stir with a rubber spatula.

5. Cover the square pan with baking parchment.

6. Pour the mixture into a square mold.

7. Chill in the refrigerator more than 4 hours or overnight.

8. Remove the mixture from the mold.

9. Cut the mixture into square pieces of 1.5 cm x 1.5 cm*

10. Sprinkle Matcha on chocolates.

* Use hot knife to prevent sticking.

Matcha Ciccolata Rojo

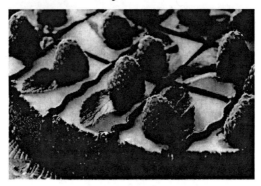

Ingredients:

(2 persons) (Makes 30 small chocolates sized 1.5cm x 1.5cm x 1.5cm)

10ml cream	150 g white chocolate
5 g butter	1 tablespoon dried red fruit (3 g)

1 tablespoon of Matcha to mix with chocolate (3 g)

1 tablespoon dried red fruit for sprinkling (3 g)

Preparation:

1. Heat the cream in a small saucepan over medium heat.

2. Crush white chocolate and put it into the cream and melt, stirring.

3. Add 3 g Matcha and stir with a rubber spatula until smooth.

4. Crush berries and stir with a rubber spatula.

5. Cover the square pan, 10cm x 10cm, with baking parchment.

6. Pour the mixture into a square mold.

7. Chill in the refrigerator more than 4 hours or overnight.

8. Remove the mixture from the mold.

9. Cut into square pieces of 1.5 cm x 1.5 cm.*

10. Serve cut chocolates on the plate and sprinkle crushed berries.

* Use hot knife to prevent sticking.

Daifuki Matcha

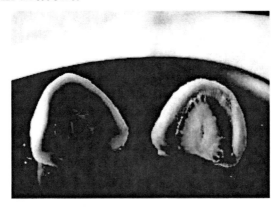

Ingredients:

150 g rice flour (shiratamako)   200 g of white bean paste

180 g of water   2 teaspoons of Matcha green tea

70 g sugar   8 strawberries

Small amount of potato starch (katakuriko)

Preparation:

1. In a bowl, dissolve Matcha with a little water.

2. Mix Matcha with white bean paste.

3. Cover strawberries with the pasta.

4. Mix rice flour, sugar, and water.

5. Put the mixture in the microwave and heat for 2 minutes (600w).

6. Mix it quickly with a wooden spoon.

7. Heat again and mix again and repeat until it becomes almost transparent.

8. Spread potato starch on a plate.

9. Extend Mochi and divide it into 8 pieces.

10. Cover strawberry with mochi paste and make round shape.

Green Cookies

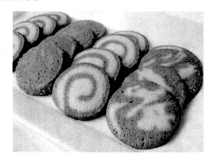

Ingredients:

(for 30 cookies, 5mm thick)

360 g flour   2 eggs

130 g sugar   1 egg yolk

240 g butter at room temperature

2 tablespoon Matcha green tea powder

1 tablespoon of Gyokuro green tea leaves

Preparation:

1. Leave the butter out of the refrigerator to soften.

2. Shift the flour and Matcha twice (we used COOK MATCHA of The Matcha House brand).

3. In a large bowl, beat the butter. Add sugar and beat again until the texture becomes creamy.

4. Add beaten eggs and continue beating until the mixture becomes yellow-white.

5. Add flour mixture and mix slowly with a rubber spatula until dough just comes together.

6. Add Gyokuro tea leaves and mix well.

7. Pull dough in a log, approximately 4 cm in diameter.

8. Wrap dough log and place in freezer for 15 minutes.

9. Cut dough 5mm thick.

10. Bake on parchment lined baking sheets for 20 minutes at 170°C (350°F).

Matcha Pancakes

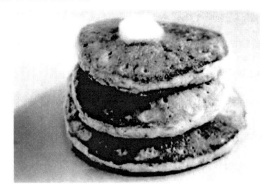

Ingredients:

150 g flour	a pinch of salt
1 egg	1 teaspoon rum
1 teaspoon baking powder	1 cup milk (120ml)
1 tablespoon sugar	2 teaspoons Matcha

Assorted toppings, such as honey, butter, maple syrup, sweetened whipped cream, or chocolate syrup. (We strongly recommend raspberry jam!)

Preparation:

1. In a bowl, mix all powders.

2. Add beaten egg, milk, and rum and whisk all together.

3. Let the pancake mix stand for at least 15 minutes before cooking.

4. Lightly grease the pan with oil.

5. It is recommended to cool down the pan slightly on a wet cloth before cooking.

6. Cook large spoonfuls of batter until bubbles burst on the surface.

7. Turn and cook other side.

8. Add toppings as you like!

Matcha Smoothie

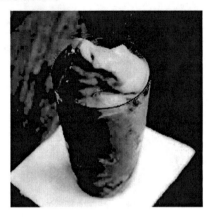

Ingredients:

1/2 of a banana

200ml of milk or soy milk

2 g of honey (one teaspoon)

2 g of Matcha (one teaspoon)

4-5 ice cubes

Put all ingredients into a mixer and mix 1 minute.

Matcha Croissant

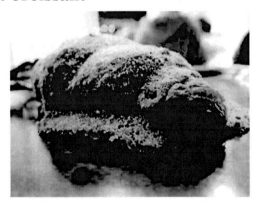

After toasting your croissant in the morning, add a pinch of Matcha powder to the top.

Matcha Cereal

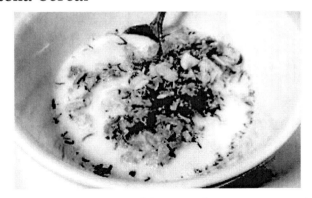

Add Matcha to any breakfast cereal or yogurt to enjoy its amazing effect.

Matcha Ochazuke

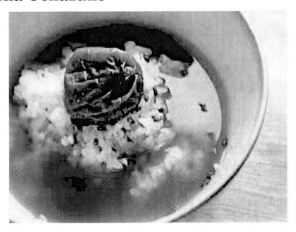

Ingredients:

1 cup of cooked white rice   Seaweed, a pinch

1/2 teaspoon of salt   Hot Genmaicha Tea 150ml

1/2 teaspoon of Matcha   Umeboshi 1 unit

1 teaspoon of Kombucha powder

Roasted glutinous rice or crispy rice cracker

How to prepare (for one serving):

1. Put hot cooked white rice in a bowl.

2. Put salt, rice crackers, Kombucha powder, and Matcha powder on the rice.

3. Add one Umeboshi.

4. Prepare hot Genmaicha tea.

5. Pour hot tea on the rice.

6. Add cut seaweed.

Matcha Curry

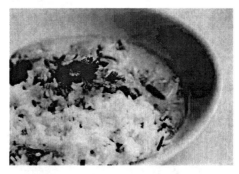

For Curry:

200g skinless chicken breast	2 bouillon cubes
2 tbsp sunflower oil	1 piece of laurel
1 carrot	Salt
1 chopped large onion	Pepper
1 tbsp minced ginger	1 tbsp of honey
2 minced garlic cloves	150ml of cream
2 tbsp of curry powder	1 tablespoon Matcha
300ml water	Cilantro

For Rice:

(quantity for cooking with rice cooking machine)

300g rice (blend of long grain rice, steamed rice, red rice, and long black rice)

400ml water

Preparation of curry:

1. Finely chop the onion. Cut the carrot and the chicken into small pieces too.

2. In a saucepan, heat oil and cook onion and carrot until the onion becomes transparent.

3. Add chicken, garlic and ginger. Cook 5 minutes more, stirring occasionally.

4. Add water, bouillon cubes, curry powder, and honey and cook for 15 minutes.

5. Turn off and, then, add cream and Matcha and mix well. Add salt and pepper and change the flavor as you like. Heat, again, for another 5 minutes.

6. Serve curry over hot rice and decorate with cilantro or parsley.

As you can see, there are many more ways to consume Matcha rather than in its beverage form. Hopefully, this will give you some inspiration and assist you in moving forward with your own creations.

There is little doubt of the importance of drinking Matcha. The science simply does not lie. Drinking Matcha is a solution that will pay dividends for years to come for better health. I hope you will take this on as a new life habit. Please share any thoughts you may have about Matcha tea with me. You can find me at http://www.matchapedia.com. Drink Matcha every day. Sip slowly and remember to slow the world around you while you enjoy the delicious benefits of Matcha tea.

Chapter 10: Essential Science of Tea

Everything you ever wanted to know about tea in about 15 pages

For centuries, tea has arguably been one of the most widely popular beverages in the entire world. In fact, one might even go ahead and argue that tea comes in second only to water, and perhaps only beating out coffee as one of the most beloved brews in history. Almost all tea comes to us from an evergreen bush known as *Camellia sinensis*. It's found all over the world but is most readily available in Asian, tropical, and subtropical parts of the world. What's great about the *C. sinensis* is that it's not limited to only making green or black tea. In fact, other teas, like your English breakfast tea, white tea, oolong, Earl Grey, and orange pekoe tea, can also be made from this versatile little bush.

Tea is celebrated the world over for a variety of reasons and has been for more years than anybody can remember. It's more than likely that tea was even used in prehistoric times, but there is quite obviously no way of knowing this for sure. What we do know is that people have been enjoying the benefits of tea for centuries, and the more we're able to accomplish with science, the more we are able to understand about tea and exactly how beneficial it really is. We'll talk a little bit about the history and composition about tea so that we can cultivate a better understanding about how this wonderful drink can potentially enrich our lives and also know a little something about how it goes about doing so.

A Brief History of Tea

Most likely, tea has its origins in Southeast Asia; the first recorded instance of tea-drinking is certainly debatable. Of course, everything popular has a creation myth, and tea is no exception. One of the interesting stories about the creation of tea involves one of China's earliest emperors, who went by the name of Shen Nung. He was the scientific sort and was really excited about experimenting with different herbs and seeing what kinds of effects they had on his constitution and health. He also happened to be extremely fascinated with boiling his water before he drank it. The story goes that one day as he was doing this a tea leaf fell into the pot. He tasted the brew, thoroughly enjoyed the way it made him feel, and tea was born.

An even more colorful creation story for tea gives it something of a practical point of origin and involves a Buddhist monk trying to meditate. Anyone familiar with meditation knows that it involves deep states of relaxation, but nobody wants to fall asleep whilst trying to attain spiritual enlightenment. One story goes that the monk, Bodhidharam, had been meditating for so long that he fell asleep. In order to make sure this didn't happen again, he took the rather extreme measure of cutting off his eyelids. They fell to the ground and transformed into the tea plant, which in turn helped him to stay awake during his meditation.

We may never know which story about the origin of tea is actually true, but we do know that the records of tea's cultivation started showing up right around the fourth century in China. By the time the 8th century had arrived, the drinking of tea had spread to Japan, and its popularity was increasing rapidly. It was right around this time that the *Ch'a Ching* arrived. Written and illustrated by Lu Yu, and spanning three volumes, it was a comprehensive guide to

As the 1500s arrived, tea had spread to Europe thanks to the Venetians and their trading routes. Everybody was pretty crazy about tea, and most of Europe set about figuring out how they could get more of it. At first, the English and the Dutch went about getting their tea by sea, while the Russians went by land to get as much of the stuff as they could. By the 1800s, tea had become an incredibly huge part of the culture. It had begun its life as a breakfast drink before becoming adopted as a more afternoon-oriented tradition. It's safe to say that between 1700 and 1800 tea importation to Britain increased a thousand fold. Eventually the Europeans wanted to go ahead and control more of the tea trade; the British established tea plantations throughout India, while the Dutch put theirs in Indonesia.

These days, almost everyone in the world drinks tea. Black is perhaps the most popular type, with green tea being favored mostly throughout Asian cultures. There are a lot of reasons for its widespread popularity; its uses are varied, and the compounds within it can be applied to a number of products. Taking a closer look at the compounds that go into tea make it easy to understand why its benefits are so widely appreciated.

What's in Tea?

Tea is as valuable as it is, in terms of health, because of the presence of *polyphenolic compounds*. These are basically referred to as flavonoids and polyphenols—both of which are *antioxidants*. You've almost certainly heard this word in the recent past, as it's become one of the most popular dietary buzzwords in recent memory. While antioxidants are actually quite good for your body (you will produce them naturally, whether you drink tea or not), they are not the wonder-substance that many marketing executives might have you believe they are. It helps to understand a bit more about the antioxidants in tea and exactly how they function.

In green tea, there are four main polyphenolic compounds (which also happen to be a type of flavonoid called a *catechin*) that give the drink its many health advantages. *Epigallocatechin-3-gallate* is probably the most popular and is commonly referred to as EGCG. *Epicatechin-3-gallate* (ECG), *epigallocatechin* (EGC), and *epicatechin* (EC) are the other main polyphenolic compounds in green tea. There are fewer of these compounds found in black teas because they have a tendency to become part of larger compounds during the process through which black tea is made. Both types of tea have fluoride, with more being found in older leaves and less in younger ones. Another trait common to both types is the fact that caffeine content is variable and mostly depends on the chemical makeup of the leaf, combined with the brewing time, grade, and size of the leaves. Often black tea is thought to have roughly twice the caffeine as green tea, but this has been seen to be untrue on numerous occasions.

So How Does It All Work?

Currently, scientists are actually still on their way to understanding a lot about how the compounds found in tea actually go about working their magic. At this point, we know that tea does a lot of good things, even if we don't necessarily know *how* it goes about doing those amazing things. For instance, one of the things that we know is that tea can help with the ability to process information, at least for a short amount of time. This was shown in a clinical study during which test subjects were given a series of tests.[1]

Of course, this benefit is most likely the result of caffeine[2], which is also found in other drinks. While many of the benefits that tea offers are unique to tea, a lot of them are still not fully understood by scientists. These compounds have shown themselves to be helpful to us in a lot of ways, but they also behave in certain ways that we don't quite understand. Nevertheless, these helpful compounds are added to a host of other products, from chewing gum to cereal and toothpaste.

The flavonoids and polyphenols found in tea are the chemical compounds that wind up giving us the most benefit. These are typically antioxidants, which means that they go about eliminating free radicals from your body. You've undoubtedly seen numerous food labels shouting about how wonderful antioxidants are but might be wondering exactly what it is they do. They put a stop to a process called oxidative stress, which basically causes the cells in your body to die. Of course, this process is an important part of many functions, exercise being chief among them. The oxidative stress that comes after a good workout is often attributed to muscle growth. In many cases, however, this oxidative stress isn't desired. The flavonoids in green tea and the polyphenols in black tea are naturally-occurring compounds that go about getting rid of these free radicals in your body. They also prevent iron from producing free radicals by binding to its molecules inside your body. This, of course, will actually negate the purpose of iron supplements, so it's smart not to mix tea with iron supplements if you need to take them.

The free radicals that result from a compound known as nitric oxide can actually cause cancer, which is one of the reasons that tea is thought to be so beneficial. To a degree, your body actually needs nitric oxide. Too much, however, is bad for you. This compound is important in that it helps to keep your blood pressure low and helps with inflammation. When nitric oxide reacts with something known as superoxide, however, it can bind with proteins and enter into a process known as nitrosylation. This process leads to the formation of cancerous cells but is actually halted, in most cases, by the antioxidants that are found within tea.

Interestingly enough, this is not *always* how these antioxidants function. In fact, the flavonoids in green tea have been seen doing exactly the opposite and bringing about oxidative stress instead of preventing it. This can create dangerous compounds in your body that will damage your DNA. The catechins that are found in green tea, however, will bring about something known as *apoptosis*. This is a form of "cellular suicide," and tea's compounds are able to create this reaction in cancer cells.

Another way that tea works to fight cancer is through the compound known as EGCG. What's interesting about this compound is that it has a tendency to destroy cancerous cells while acting as an antioxidant that helps with cell growth at other times. Since this catechin can act as an antioxidant at certain times and can destroy cells at other times, it can theoretically both help and hinder the growth of cancerous cells. Tea is obviously not any kind of significant carcinogen, and tests performed on animals have shown very positive results when it comes to tea's ability to fight cancer. Typically, it's shown that green tea is better for cancer than black tea[3], but this could easily have something to do with the fact that more studies surrounding tea's effects upon cancer have been focused on green tea. When it comes down to it, though, animal studies have shown positive results when it comes to tea's ability to fight cancer in over eighty significant studies that have looked at multiple types of cancer, including (but certainly not limited to) stomach, throat, colon, pancreas, bladder, and many others.[4]

Another way that tea helps the human body relates to something known as the P53 gene. This is an important part of your genetic makeup, as it helps to make sure that tumors don't get very far, if and when they start to grow. When a tumor pops up, your P53 gene activates and makes sure that the tumor isn't allowed to

Matcha Green Tea

continue growing. Cancerous developments are stopped in their tracks this way, but things like colon cancer are a lot more likely when this gene doesn't work well. What's nice, however, is that tea stimulates this gene's activity. When your P53 gene spots a tumor starting to grow, it will either freeze that cell in mid-division or cause it to kill itself via apoptosis. Tea also acts to inhibit your AP-1 protein. This actually isn't a good thing if you're trying to do something like heal a wound, but when it comes to the development of cancerous cells, this can actually be quite handy.

The compound EGCG also helps to inhibit something called angiogenesis. This is a word that describes the development of brand new capillaries within your body. Again, when you're trying to heal a wound, this is something that your body quite desperately needs. In the event that you're dealing with a tumor, however, the inhibition of angiogenesis can be great for making sure things don't get too cancerous. In fact, there is even a theory that angiogenesis inhibitors can help prevent fat cells by getting more blood, but this is going to need a bit more research.

Much lab work has been done to determine whether or not compounds found in tea help with weight loss in a significant way. While we're still trying to understand more about how this might work, it's been found that EGCG can help to inhibit digestive enzymes, at least in mice. The testing done on humans didn't fare quite as well, but testing done on mice showed that EGCG was causing calories to pass right through the mice without being digested (essentially the same thing that happens when a human experiences diarrhea).[5] Despite the fact that this method of weight loss hasn't been clinically proven, dietary supplements are often stuffed full of EGCG, and their labels are covered with the compound's name.

Theanine is another one of tea's most important ingredients, and it helps to deprive cancer cells of a protective compound known as glutathione. This amino acid is unique to tea and resembles something called glutamate which is naturally more abundant in your body. Glutamate is a part of a compound known as glutathione, which is present in most of your cells and helps with detox and protects against all kinds of cell death and degeneration. Researchers were seeing that, in mice, cancer was being kept under control because theanine from tea was being converted to glutamate in their livers. This extra glutamate leads to more glutathione, which means less oxidative stress and other maladies. In cancer patients, this is a risky treatment, because it can actually wind up *helping* tumors; more needs to be understood before it becomes a readily-used solution.

Fluoride is something that we've all heard of, and it's actually present in most of the tea that you drink. In fact, it's actually cheaper tea that has higher amounts of fluoride and for a very interesting reason. Cheaper tea has a tendency to be made from older leaves, but these ones have accumulated the most fluoride, which is great for your bones and your teeth. Most of the time, tea gets its fluoride through something known as bioaccumulation, wherein it absorbs this material through the soil. Typically this happens with things like pesticides and other toxic compounds, but in tea, the absorption of fluoride actually gives it the ability to fight against osteoporosis. Both types of tea (green and black) will help with this, but based on studies conducted over the course of about 10 years, it was shown that green tea has a greater effect[6] than black tea[7].

Yet another great benefit that comes with the drinking of a lot of tea is the prevention of Parkinson's disease. Of course, this is attributed to daily caffeine consumption, but this is something that can certainly be accomplished with tea. Of course, decaf tea can give you a lot of the other benefits that come along with this wonderful brew if you don't like the jittery feeling that can often accompany caffeine. Caffeine works its magic by preventing a molecule called adenosine from sticking to receptors that are located in your brain. Throughout the day, this molecule will build up as a result of your energy output. When there are enough of them, they bind to the receptors in your brain, and you get tired. Caffeine prevents this from happening. In fact, this is actually how caffeine prevents Parkinson's disease, which is brought on when nerve cells that produce dopamine start to die. While we don't know exactly what causes this to happen, we do know that the dopamine-boosting effects of caffeine help to prevent Parkinson's.[8] What's interesting is that this was actually shown to be dependent on the dosage involved in the experiment when men were the subject but not for women.[9, 10]

Caffeine can also help you out with your headache, by causing your blood vessels to open up in some places (like your lungs and muscles), while constricting them in others (like your skin and your brain). A lot of headaches, in fact, are associated with dilated blood vessels in your brain, which is why a lot of over-the-counter headache medicines have caffeine in them. Next time, try some tea instead of a pill; you might be surprised at the result!

Tannin is another compound found in tea, and it can help you relieve things like puffy skin and diarrhea. It's found in both green and black tea, and it can help your skin by binding to protein molecules and shrinking them. This helps to make your tissue tighten and can reduce puffiness. Tannin can also coat the inside of your stomach and mitigate the things that cause diarrhea. Too much of it, however, will seriously irritate your stomach. This can be mitigated by milk.

The Good and the Bad

As you can see, tea is a pretty great thing—but it's definitely best when it's enjoyed in moderation. Especially when you're considering caffeinated tea, you want to make sure you're enjoying your favorite beverage in moderation. Even decaf tea can still have tannin that will upset your stomach. It's also smart to avoid taking iron or copper supplements with tea, as tea will negate their effects.

Folic acid is also important if your diet is high in tea, as there is some evidence that suggests that tea might interfere with the actions of this B vitamin. This vitamin moderates your homocysteine levels, which can cause cardiovascular disease and stroke if they get too high. While tea is mostly a cardiovascular protector, it can interfere with vitamin B's job, so folic acid will help you to keep your homocysteine down.

Interestingly enough, the age of the leaf will cause the components of the tea to vary in a pretty significant way. As mentioned, more expensive tea tends to come from younger buds, which also have the most caffeine, catechins, and flavonoids. They also, however, have the least fluoride.

How Is Tea Made?

Almost all tea (with the exception of herbal teas, as previously stated) is made from the leaves of an evergreen bush called *Camellia sinensis*. Interestingly enough, *C. sinensis* is actually an herb, which makes the "herbal tea" distinction an interesting one indeed. Naturally-occurring flavonoid molecules called catechins (EGCG and the other compounds we talked about so much) are positively packed into the tea leaves that go into your favorite brew, and these compounds are the source of all those goodies that help you stay healthy and fight things like cancer and weight gain.

In just about every case, the tea leaves are first dried and rolled. This is an important process, as it helps to make sure that the tea leaves don't give off their vital compounds too quickly when you steep them to actually brew your drink. Also, fresh leaves that haven't been dried will result in a brew that is weak and watery, at best. The rolling of the tea leaves is also important in that it helps the catechins mix with a certain type of enzyme known as polyphenol oxidase. This helps the catechins to form larger, more complex molecules. This process, interestingly enough, is typically referred to as "fermentation," even though microbes aren't exactly involved. Really, this process is similar to oxidization—the same thing that happens to your tea is what happens to an apple or avocado if it's exposed to the open air for too long (it turns brown in color). Since black tea is fermented, it actually has a lower catechin content. This is because those catechins polymerize into other compounds that hope to create theaflavic acid. This is the compound that gives black tea its distinctive colors and flavors. Green tea isn't fermented, because it's steamed before it's rolled. This process actually destroys the enzymes that make black tea look and taste the way it does so that fermentation doesn't occur. White tea, which has become popular for its perception as something of a status symbol, has become a lot more popular in recent years, though it hasn't been shown to be necessarily more effective than other types of tea.

Other Helpful Uses

Many believe that drinking tea can be very helpful for improving the quality of life for people with cancer and illness stemming from oxidative stress. In addition to smaller things like the cognitive boosts many claim they can get from the caffeine, there are numerous other great benefits that can come with the regular drinking of tea. A great example of other types of teas and their benefits is that studies now show that black tea can help with kidney stones (green tea is as yet untested in this regard). A study that questioned over 81,000 women found that eight percent of them saw a reduction in their kidney stones as a result of being tea drinkers.[11]

The compounds and extracts that can be pulled out of green tea have been positively packed into a variety of weight loss products, diet pills, and the like. Consumers often readily believe that these compounds treat obesity, but this hasn't necessarily been proven yet. In fact, there have been different studies performed that have shown different results. One such study didn't really see any effects when people took a green tea extract for three straight months.[12] Another saw close to a 5% reduction in both weight and waist circumference.[13] It is important to mention that these studies were done using tea extracts in many cases and that Matcha tea may have yielded different results.

While tea might not be the obesity-buster that some diet products might want you to believe people swear by it and often my friends tell me that it is the only thing that helped them take the pounds off and keep them off. Otherwise it has certainly been found to help you out with your cholesterol. There are two types of cholesterol: the "good" kind (HDL) and the "bad" kind (LDL). Green tea that was enriched with theaflavin (something black tea always has) was shown to help hypercholesterolemic test subjects decrease their LDL cholesterol levels.[14] Interestingly enough, studies found that Japanese men saw the most benefits from green tea when it comes to cholesterol.[15] Another great benefit that comes with tea is a little help for your cardiovascular system. Black tea can seriously help with a condition called atherosclerosis[16] and reduced heart attacks in individuals that drank it regularly.[17]

As you can see, tea is a pretty wonderful thing. Of course, there are the old English advertisements that proclaim it to be a wonder beverage that will "removeth lassitude" and "vanquish heavy dreams,"[18] but those are a bit of a stretch. In reality, though, most doctors can agree tea has a ton of great benefits that you can enjoy when you include it in your daily diet.

References:

1. I. Hindmarch, P.T. Quinlan, K.L. Moore, and C. Parkin, "The effects of black tea and other beverages on aspects of cognition and psychomotor performance," *Psychopharmacology* (Berl) 1998 Oct; 139(3): 230-38.

2. P.J. Durlach, "The effects of a low dose of caffeine on cognitive performance," *Psychofarmacology* (Berl) 1998 Nov; 140(1): 116-19.

3. C. S. Yang, J. Chung, G. Yang, S.K. Chabra, and M.J. Lee, "Tea and tea polyphenols in cancer prevention," *J Nutr* 2000 Feb; 130(25 Suppl): 472S-478S.

4. F.L. Chung, J. Schwartz, C.R. Hertzog, and Y.M. Yang, "Tea and cancer prevention, studies in animals and humans," *J Nutr* 2003 Oct; 133(10): 3268S-3274S.

5. S. Klaus, S. Pultz, C. Thone-Reineke, and S. Wolfram, "Epigallocatechin gallate attenuates diet-induced obesity in mice by decreasing energy absorption and increasing fat oxidation," *Int J Obes Relat Metab Disord*.

6. C.H. Wu, Y.C. Yang, W.J. Yao, J.S. Wu, C.J. Chang, "Epidemiological evidence of increased bone mineral density in habitual tea drinkers," *Arch Intern Med* 2002, May 13; 162(9): 1001-06.

7. Z. Chen, M.B. Pettinger, C. Ritenbaugh, A.Z. LaCroix, J. Robbins, B.J. Caan, D.H. Barad, and I.A. Hakim, "Habitual tea consumption and risk of osteoporosis: a prospective study in the women's health initiative observational cohort," *Am J Epidemiol* 2003 Oct 15; 158(8): 772-81.

8. G.W. Ross, R.D. Abbott, H. Petrovitch, D.M. Morens, A. Grandinetti, K.H. Tung, C.M. Tanner, K.H. Masaki, P.L. Blanchette, J.D. Curb, J.S. Popper, and L.R. White, "Association of coffee and caffeine intake with the risk of Parkinson's disease," *JAMA* 2000 May 24-31; 283(20): 2674-79.

9. E.K. Tan, C. Tan, S.M. Fook-Chong, S.Y. Lum, A. Chai, H. Chung, H. Shen, Y. Zhao, M.L. Teoh, Y. Yih, R. Pavanni, V.R. Chandran, M.C. Wong, "Dose-dependant protective effect of

coffee, tea, and smoking in Parkinson's disease: a study in ethnic Chinese," *J Neurol Sci* 2003 Dec 15; 216(1): 163-67.

10. A. Ascherio, S.M. Zhang, M.A. Hernan, I. Kawachi, G.A. Colditz, F.E. Speizer, and W.C. Willett, "Prospective study of caffeine consumption, and risk of Parkinson's disease in men and women," *Ann Neurol*, 2001 July; 501(1): 56-63.

11. G.C. Curhan, W.C. Willett, F.E. Speizer, M.J. Stampfer, "Beverage use and risk for kidney stones in women," *Ann Intern Med* 1998 April 1; 128(7): 534-40.

12. E.M. Kovacs, M.P. Lejeune, I. Nijs, M.S. Westerterp-Plantenga, "Effects of green tea on weight maintenance after body-weight loss," *Br J Nutr* 2004 Mar; 91(3): 431-37.

13. P. Chantre and D. Lairon, "Recent findings of green tea extract AR25 (Exolise) and its activity for the treatment of obesity," *Phytomedicine* 2002 Jan; 9(1): 3-8.

14. D.J. Maron, G.P. Lu, N.S. Cai, Z.G. Wu, Y.H. Li, H. Chen, J.Q. Zhu, X.J. Jin, B.C. Wouters, and J. Zhao, "Cholesterol lowering effects of a theaflavin-enriched green tea extract: a randomized controlled trial," *Arch Intern Med* 2003 June 23; 163(12): 1448-53.

15. K. Imai, and K. Nakachi, "Cross-sectional study of effects of drinking green tea on cardiovascular and liver diseases," *BMJ*, 1995 Mar 18; 310(6981): 693-96.

16. J.M. Geleijnse, L.J. Launer, A. Hofman, H.A. Pols, and J.C. Witterman, "Tea flavonoids may protect against atherosclerosis: the Rotterdam study," *Arch Intern Med* 1999 Oct 11; 159(18): 2170-74.

17. J.M. Geleijnse, L.J. Launer, D.A. Van der Kuip, A. Hofman, and J.C. Witterman, "Inverse association of tea and flavonoid intakes with incident myocardial infarction: the Rotterdam Study," *Am J Clin Nutr* 2002 May; 75(5): 880-86.

18. J.H. Hui, *Encyclopedia of Food Science and Technology* (New York: John Wiley, 1992).

Index

Matcha Green Tea

Matcha Green Tea

References:

- Green tea. Natural Medicines Comprehensive Database Web site. Accessed at www.naturaldatabase.com on July 8, 2009.

- Green tea (*Camellia sinensis*). Natural Standard Database Web site. Accessed at www.naturalstandard.com on July 8, 2009.

- National Cancer Institute. *Tea and Cancer Prevention*. Strengths and Limits of the Evidence. National Cancer Institute Web site. Accessed   at www.cancer.gov/cancertopics/factsheet/prevention/tea on June 3, 2010.

- Sarma DN, Barrett ML, Chavez ML, et al. Safety of green tea extracts: a systematic review by the US Pharmacopeia. *Drug Safety*. 2008;31(6):469–484.

- Yanyan Wang, Maoquan Li, Xueqing Xu, Min Song, Huansheng Tao, Yun Bai. **Green tea epigallocatechin-3-gallate (EGCG) promotes neural progenitor cell proliferation and sonic hedgehog pathway activation during adult hippocampal neurogenesis.** *Molecular Nutrition & Food Research*, 2012; 56 (8): 1292 DOI: 10.1002/mnfr.201200035

- U. Heinrich, et al. Green tea polyphenols provide photoprotection, increase microcirculation, and modulate skin properties of women. Journal of Nutrition Doi: 10.3945/jn.110.136465.
  free   abstract   : http://jn.nutrition.org/content/early/2011/04/27/jn.110.136465.abstract

- 17. Hara, Yukihiko. Green tea: health benefits and applications. Vol. 106. CRC, 2001.

About the Author

Shaahin Cheyene

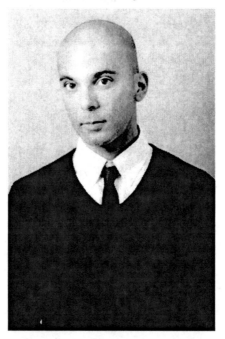

Shaahin Cheyene is the CEO and Chairman of brain nutrition start-up, Accelerated Intelligence. Cheyene shares his passion to accelerate intelligence through his latest company and products.

Born in Iran, Shaahin Cheyene is an award-winning entrepreneur, writer, and filmmaker currently based in Los Angeles, California. In the early 1990s, while still in his teens, Cheyene spearheaded the "Smart Drug Movement" by inventing and branding the original Herbal Ecstasy and over 200 other award-winning products.

CPSIA information can be obtained at www.ICGtesting.com
Printed in the USA
LVOW10s0108081015

457411LV00027B/508/P

9 781482 623239